Anatomy & Physiology for Complete Beginners

The Definitive Guide to Mastering the Basics of Human Anatomy and Physiology On How the Body's Structure Maintains Balance and Health and Enables Function

Mina Mong
Copyright@2024

TABLE OF CONTENT

CHAPTER 1 3
    INTRODUCTION 3
CHAPTER 2 10
    Overview of Human Anatomy 10
CHAPTER 3 18
    The Musculoskeletal System 18
CHAPTER 4 26
    The Nervous System 26
CHAPTER 5 34
    The Circulatory System 34
CHAPTER 6 41
    The Respiratory System 41
CHAPTER 7 48
    The Digestive System 48
CHAPTER 8 55
    The Urinary System 55
CHAPTER 9 62
    The Endocrine System 62
CHAPTER 10 68
    The Immune System 68
CHAPTER 11 75
    The Integumentary System 75
CHAPTER 12 82
    The Reproductive System 82
THE END 88

CHAPTER 1

INTRODUCTION

Objective of the Manual
The human body showcases an extraordinary level of complexity, featuring intricately linked systems that collaborate seamlessly to sustain life. This guide aims to offer a clear and thorough introduction to the fundamentals of human anatomy and physiology, tailored for those who are just starting out and have minimal prior knowledge. This guide is designed for students, health enthusiasts, or anyone with a curiosity about the workings of the body, providing a clear understanding of the essential concepts of anatomy and physiology.

Summary of Human Structure and Function
The study of anatomy focusses on the organisation and structure of the body and its components—exploring what constitutes the body and how these elements are arranged. Physiology, conversely, examines the mechanisms by which these structures operate to maintain life. Comprehending anatomy without physiology resembles being familiar with the components of a car while lacking insight into its operation; conversely, exploring physiology without anatomy is comparable to grasping the car's mechanics without recognising the specific mechanical elements involved.

This guide seeks to illustrate the interconnectedness of structure and function in living organisms. By comprehending both, you will gain a more precise understanding of how the body's structures play a role in its overall functioning.

- What Is the Significance of Anatomy?
The study of anatomy provides a profound understanding of how the human body is structured, ranging from the intricate details of cells to the comprehensive layout of the whole organism. It elucidates the structure that underpins existence, encompassing the skeletal system, musculature, organs, and tissues that form the body's design.

- What Is the Significance of Physiology?
The study of physiology uncovers the intricate mechanisms enabling the body's structures to perform vital functions like respiration, digestion, and locomotion. It describes the processes by which our bodies transform food into energy, defend against illnesses, and facilitate communication between the brain and other bodily systems.

In unison, anatomy and physiology elucidate the "what" and "how" of the body's functions, providing a comprehensive insight into the intricacies of human life.

Significance of Grasping the Mechanisms of the Body
What is the significance of understanding anatomy and physiology for someone just starting out? This knowledge offers numerous practical and intellectual benefits that go well beyond simple curiosity.

1. Individual Health and Wellness
Understanding the mechanisms of your body empowers you to make educated choices regarding your well-being. It enables you to grasp the reasons behind the effectiveness of various diets, the effects of exercise on different bodily systems, and the mechanisms by which

medical treatments or medications operate. Gaining insight into the processes occurring within your body enables you to provide it with more effective care.

2. Avoidance of Disease

Grasping fundamental physiological concepts enables you to identify potential issues within your body. For instance, understanding the workings of your circulatory system allows you to grasp the importance of high blood pressure and the measures you can implement to avert it. Understanding the immune system allows for a clearer interpretation of vaccinations, infections, and strategies for disease prevention.

3. Analytical Reasoning in Health Care

Whether you are keen on a career in the life sciences or simply wish to enhance your knowledge as a patient, studying anatomy and physiology can enrich your comprehension of biological concepts. You will be more prepared to participate in discussions with healthcare experts, pose pertinent enquiries, and evaluate medical information with a discerning eye.

4. Everyday Operations and Bodily Consciousness

The human body serves as the essential instrument for engaging with the environment. Grasping its mechanisms can enhance your appreciation for its abilities and constraints. You'll cultivate an understanding of the significance of rest, hydration, nutrition, and mental well-being, all of which play a crucial role in achieving peak performance.

5. Delving into the Intriguing Intricacies of Existence

Lastly, studying anatomy and physiology provides insight into the complex structure of living beings. The intricate cells that serve as the foundation of life, along with the sophisticated interactions among organs and systems, showcase the remarkable design of the human body.

Intended Readers: Absolute Newcomers
This guide is tailored for individuals who are just beginning their exploration of the topic. This guide is designed for everyone, whether you're a high school student, a healthcare trainee, or just someone with a curiosity about the human body, and it requires no previous understanding. Our aim is to clarify each idea in straightforward, accessible language while steering clear of complex terminology. The material will be delivered in a systematic manner, beginning with fundamental ideas and slowly advancing to more intricate discussions.

The Interconnection Between Structure and Function in Organisms
The fundamental concept of human anatomy and physiology lies in the close connection between structure and function. Every structure in the body, ranging from the tiniest cell to the largest organ, possesses a distinct form that enables it to carry out a specific function. This connection is what enables the human body to function as a unified, living entity.

The Relationship Between Structure and Function
In the exploration of anatomy and physiology, a consistent observation emerges: the configuration of every body part is exquisitely tailored to fulfil its specific role. This idea is referred to as the form-function relationship.

Illustrations of the Connection Between Structure and Function in the Body
1. Skeletal Structure and Locomotion

The human skeleton consists of sturdy bones that offer the body essential structure and support. However, bones are not merely rigid, unchanging structures; they are formed in configurations that facilitate motion. The elongated structures in your limbs function as levers, enabling movement such as walking, running, lifting, and handling various objects. Joints, such as the ball-and-socket joint found in the shoulder, are structured to allow extensive movement, whereas the hinge joint in the elbow restricts motion to one plane, enhancing stability and strength.

2. Muscles and Force Production
Muscles consist of fibres capable of both contraction and relaxation. The arrangement of these fibres within various muscle groups plays a crucial role in determining the force they can exert and the types of movements they are capable of producing. For example, the muscles in your calves are designed for strong, repetitive actions like walking and running, whereas the muscles in your hands are more precisely adapted for tasks requiring dexterity and accuracy, such as typing or playing an instrument.

3. The Cardiovascular System and Haemodynamics
The heart is a specialised muscular organ, intricately structured to facilitate the circulation of blood throughout the body. The structure of its chambers is meticulously designed to propel blood into the major arteries with significant force, while the valves play a crucial role in maintaining unidirectional flow, effectively preventing any backflow. This anatomical feature allows the heart to sustain a consistent and rhythmic flow of blood, ensuring the delivery of oxygen and nutrients to cells while facilitating the removal of waste products.

4. The Respiratory System and Its Role in Gas Exchange

The structure of the lungs is optimised to enhance the effectiveness of gas exchange. Their porous structure and extensive surface area facilitate the diffusion of oxygen into the bloodstream, while simultaneously allowing for the expulsion of carbon dioxide. The tiny air sacs, known as alveoli, are designed to optimise this process, allowing the body to effectively take in oxygen and expel waste gases.

Significance of Equilibrium in Sustaining Well-Being
While anatomy and physiology provide insight into the harmonious arrangement of the body's structures and functions, another essential concept is homeostasis, the organism's capacity to sustain internal equilibrium.

The body strives to maintain a state of equilibrium, adapting to external fluctuations to achieve balance. The ongoing observation and adjustment of factors like temperature, pH levels, blood pressure, and glucose levels is essential. In the absence of homeostasis, the body cannot operate effectively, and even minor disruptions can result in health issues or disease.

Mechanisms of Homeostasis 1. Feedback Loops
The organism employs feedback mechanisms—both enhancing and inhibiting—to maintain its internal equilibrium. A negative feedback loop serves to counterbalance alterations within the body, facilitating a return to homeostasis. For instance, when there is an increase in body temperature, the sweat glands become active to facilitate cooling, helping to restore a stable internal temperature. Positive feedback loops serve to enhance changes, exemplified in childbirth, where contractions escalate until the baby is delivered.

2. Function of Hormones and the Nervous System

The endocrine and nervous systems are essential for the regulation of homeostasis. Insulin plays a crucial role in regulating blood sugar levels, whereas the nervous system is essential for maintaining body temperature, heart rate, and various other vital functions. These systems engage in continuous communication to maintain the body's equilibrium.

Instances of Homeostasis in Practice 1. Thermal Regulation

In a warm environment, the body's internal regulator, situated in the hypothalamus, senses the shift in temperature. It triggers processes such as perspiration to help regulate your body temperature. On the other hand, in response to cold temperatures, the body reacts by narrowing blood vessels and producing heat via shivering.

2. Regulation of Glucose Levels

Following a meal, there is an increase in your blood glucose levels. The pancreas secretes insulin, facilitating the absorption of glucose by cells for energy, which in turn reduces blood sugar levels. When blood sugar levels fall below normal, the pancreas secretes a hormone known as glucagon, which instructs the liver to release stored glucose into the bloodstream.

Grasping the connection between structure and function, along with the significance of maintaining balance, is essential for exploring human anatomy and physiology. Every component of the organism is intricately structured to function in concert with the others, preserving equilibrium and safeguarding the organism's ongoing vitality and wellness. This guide will delve into these concepts further, assisting newcomers in understanding the incredible intricacies of the human body.

CHAPTER 2

Overview of Human Anatomy

Grasping the intricacies of the human body starts with the study of anatomy, laying the groundwork for understanding the organisation and operation of our biological systems. This chapter will provide an overview of the various forms of anatomy, along with the structured arrangement of the body, progressing from cells to tissues, organs, and ultimately the complete organism.

Anatomy is the branch of science that deals with the structure of organisms and their parts. It involves the study of the physical arrangement of various systems and components within living beings, providing insights into how they function and interact.

Clarification and Elucidation
The study of anatomy focusses on the physical structures that compose living organisms. The emphasis is on recognising and detailing the anatomical characteristics of the body, encompassing bones, muscles, organs, and tissues, along with their organisation and interconnections. Essentially, anatomy serves as the blueprint of the body, aiding our comprehension of the organisation and structure of its components.

The exploration of anatomy is crucial as it establishes the foundation for comprehending physiology, which investigates how those anatomical structures carry out their specific functions. Examining anatomy provides valuable knowledge about the body's structure, essential for health practitioners, learners, and those keen on grasping the organisation of the human form.

Categories of Structural Biology

The study of anatomy can be approached through various methods, influenced by the depth of detail under consideration. There are three main categories of anatomy:

1. Macroscopic Structure

Gross anatomy, often referred to as macroscopic anatomy, focusses on the examination of structures that can be observed without the aid of a microscope. This encompasses significant anatomical structures like the brain, heart, muscles, and bones. Gross anatomy is usually acquired through dissection and careful observation of the body's overall structure, serving as an essential component of medical and biological education.

- Surface Anatomy: This branch of gross anatomy examines the visible characteristics of the body and their connections to underlying structures. For instance, by analysing the surface anatomy of the chest, it is possible to identify the location of the heart and lungs underneath.
- Regional Anatomy: This method focusses on distinct areas of the body, like the head or limbs, analysing all components within those areas, including bones, muscles, nerves, and vessels.
- Systemic Anatomy: This branch of study emphasises the examination of specific organ systems, such as the cardiovascular system or the respiratory system, rather than concentrating on individual regions.

2. Cellular Structure

Microscopic anatomy, as the term implies, pertains to the examination of structures that are not visible without the aid of magnification. This encompasses cells and tissues, necessitating the use of microscopes for observation. Microscopic anatomy can be categorised into:

- Cytology: The examination of cells, which serve as the fundamental units of life. Researchers in this field analyse the intricate details of cell structure, organisation, and function, emphasising the role of various cell types in the overall operation of the body.
- Histology: The examination of tissues, which are collections of cells collaborating to execute particular functions. Histologists examine the organisation of tissues and their roles in the structure and function of organs.

3. Growth Structure
Developmental anatomy examines the transformations and growth of the body's structures from the moment of conception all the way to adulthood. This discipline focusses on the mechanisms of development, specialisation, and progression that take place over the course of life. One significant aspect of developmental anatomy is embryology, which examines the initial phases of development, from fertilisation to the creation of the foetus.

Principal Hierarchies of Structure

The human body exhibits a structured organisation, beginning with the most basic unit—the cell—and advancing through increasingly intricate formations until we arrive at the complete, functioning organism. Grasping these levels of organisation is essential, as each level is constructed upon the prior one, leading to the emergence of more intricate structures as components collaborate in increasing quantities.

1. Cells: The Fundamental Building Block of Existence
Cells represent the essential building blocks of all living organisms. These entities represent the tiniest units that can execute all essential life processes, such as metabolism, growth, and reproduction. The human body is composed of trillions of cells, each uniquely adapted to carry out essential functions crucial for its overall operation.

- Types of Cells: The human body comprises a diverse array of cells, including muscle cells, nerve cells, red blood cells, and epithelial cells. Every type possesses a distinct structure that enables it to carry out its specific function. For instance, red blood cells are specialised for the transportation of oxygen, whereas nerve cells are organised to convey electrical signals.
- Cell Architecture: Cells possess a range of components that enable them to perform their essential functions. These components consist of the nucleus, housing genetic material, the mitochondria, responsible for energy production, and the cell membrane, regulating the entry and exit of substances within the cell.

Cells operate collaboratively, forming groups that create tissues, representing the subsequent level of organisation.

2. Tissues: Collections of Cells Collaborating
A tissue consists of a collection of similar cells collaborating to execute a shared function. The human body consists of four primary types of tissues, each uniquely adapted for specific functions:

- Epithelial Tissue: This category of tissue serves to cover the surfaces of the body and line various cavities. This structure acts as a protective barrier against injury and infection, while also being involved in processes such as absorption, secretion, and sensation. Instances encompass the epidermis and the inner surface of the gastrointestinal system.
- Connective Tissue: This type of tissue plays a crucial role in supporting and linking various tissues and organs within the body. This encompasses a range of subtypes, including bone, cartilage, blood, and adipose tissue. Connective tissue plays a crucial role in providing structural support, storing energy, and facilitating the transport of substances throughout the body.
- Muscle Tissue: This type of tissue plays a crucial role in facilitating movement within organisms. Muscle tissue can be categorised into three distinct types: skeletal muscle, responsible for voluntary movements; cardiac muscle, which facilitates blood circulation through the heart; and smooth muscle, governing involuntary actions like digestion.
- Nervous Tissue: This type of tissue is uniquely adapted for the purpose of communication within the body. The structure consists of neurones that convey electrical signals and glial cells that offer essential support. Nervous tissue is located in the brain, spinal cord, and nerves, enabling the body to detect stimuli and react to alterations in the environment.

Cells come together to create tissues, which then organise into organs, representing a higher level of biological complexity.

3. Organs: Collaborative Functions of Tissues
A structure made up of two or more distinct types of tissues that collaborate to carry out a particular function is known as an organ. Every organ possesses a

distinct form and composition that aligns perfectly with its function within the organism. For instance:

- The Heart: Made up of specialised muscle tissue, supportive connective tissue, and protective epithelial tissue, the heart plays a crucial role in circulating blood throughout the organism.
- The Respiratory Organs: The lungs, composed of epithelial and connective tissues, play a crucial role in gas exchange, enabling the entry of oxygen into the bloodstream while facilitating the expulsion of carbon dioxide.
- The Stomach: Composed of layers of epithelial, muscle, and connective tissues, this organ is essential for digestion, facilitating the breakdown of food to enable nutrient absorption.

Each organ has a unique role, yet none operates independently. Organs come together to create organ systems, which work in harmony to sustain the health of the body.

4. Organ Systems: The Assembly of Organs into Functional Units
A collection of organs collaborates within an organ system to execute a wider range of functions. The human body comprises 11 major organ systems, with each system tasked with distinct functions:

- The Digestive System: Comprises the stomach, intestines, liver, and additional organs that play a crucial role in the breakdown of food and the absorption of nutrients.
- The Respiratory System: Made up of the lungs, trachea, and various components that facilitate breathing and the exchange of gases.

- The Circulatory System: Comprising the heart, blood vessels, and blood, it facilitates the movement of oxygen, nutrients, and waste products across the body.
- The Nervous System: Comprises the brain, spinal cord, and nerves, orchestrating bodily functions and reacting to external stimuli.
- The Muscular System: This system is essential for movement and encompasses skeletal muscles, cardiac muscles, and smooth muscles.
- The Skeletal System: Made up of bones, cartilage, and ligaments, it serves to provide structure and support, while also safeguarding essential organs.
- The Endocrine System: Comprising various glands such as the thyroid and adrenal glands, it oversees bodily functions by means of hormones.
- The Lymphatic and Immune System: Plays a crucial role in defending the body against pathogens and ensuring proper fluid equilibrium.
- The Urinary System: Comprises the kidneys and bladder, playing a crucial role in blood filtration and waste elimination.
- The Reproductive System: Essential for the generation of new life and the management of sexual health.
- The Integumentary System: Comprises the skin, hair, and nails, serving as a barrier and playing a crucial role in temperature regulation.

Every organ system is essential for maintaining the overall functionality of the body.

5. Entity: The Comprehensive Human Anatomy
The human body represents the pinnacle of biological organisation, functioning as a fully integrated organism. The intricate interplay of the body's organ systems collaborates seamlessly to maintain the essence of life. This intricate interplay necessitates ongoing dialogue and teamwork among cells, tissues, organs, and systems.

The primary aim of these various levels of organisation is to uphold equilibrium and well-being, allowing the organism as a complete entity to operate effectively within its surroundings.

The exploration of human anatomy encompasses the examination of the body's structure, ranging from the microscopic intricacies of cells to the macroscopic complexities of entire organ systems and the organism as a whole. Grasping these levels of organisation enhances our appreciation for the intricate nature of the human body and the collaborative function of its components in sustaining life and health.

CHAPTER 3

The Musculoskeletal System

The musculoskeletal system serves as the framework of the body, offering support and facilitating movement. This system is made up of bones, muscles, joints, tendons, and ligaments, all collaborating to facilitate movement, safeguard essential organs, and uphold posture. This chapter delves into the structure and function of the musculoskeletal system, highlighting the importance of bones as the body's framework, the various types and roles of muscles, and the crucial function of joints in facilitating movement.

Bones: The Structural Foundation of the Body

Anatomy and Physiology of Skeletal Elements
The skeletal system serves as the essential framework of the human body, offering support, safeguarding vital organs, and facilitating movement. Bones are solid, mineralised formations composed mainly of collagen, a protein that imparts strength and flexibility, along with calcium phosphate, a mineral that contributes to the bone's hardness. While they might appear to be solid structures, bones are actually dynamic, living tissues that are in a continual state of growth and repair.

The main roles of bones are as follows: - Support: Bones serve as the structural framework that upholds the body and preserves its form. In the absence of a skeletal structure, the body would be unable to maintain its form and would succumb to the pressure of its own mass.

- Protection: The skeletal structure serves to safeguard essential organs, including the brain, which is encased by the skull, as well as the heart and lungs, which are shielded by the ribcage.
- Movement: Skeletal structures function as levers, which are manipulated by muscular contractions to facilitate motion. The configuration of skeletal structures and articulations dictates the variety and extent of motion achievable.
- Mineral Storage: Bones serve as a reservoir for vital minerals, especially calcium and phosphorus, which can be mobilised into the bloodstream when required.
- Haematopoiesis: The skeletal system houses bone marrow, the site of production for erythrocytes, leukocytes, and thrombocytes.

Categories of Skeletal Structures (Elongated, Compact, Flat, etc.)
The diversity of bone shapes and sizes reflects their specialised functions within the organism. There are various classifications of bones, which encompass:

- Long Bones: These structures are characterised by their greater length compared to width and are predominantly located in the limbs. Long bones, including the femur and humerus, play a crucial role in facilitating movement and serve as levers that muscles utilise to propel the body. Bone marrow is also present, serving as the site for blood cell production.
- Short Bones: These bones are roughly equal in length and width, offering both stability and a degree of movement. The wrist bones, known as carpals, and the ankle bones, referred to as tarsals, serve as prime examples of short bones in the skeletal system.
- Flat Bones: These structures are characterised by their thin and often curved nature, serving the crucial role of safeguarding internal organs while offering a broad

surface area for the attachment of muscles. Instances encompass the skull, ribs, and sternum (breastbone).
- Irregular Bones: These bones possess intricate shapes that do not conform to the other classifications. Irregular bones, including the vertebrae and pelvis, serve crucial functions by offering support and protection, all while permitting a degree of movement.
- Sesamoid Bones: These small, rounded structures are found nestled within tendons. The patella, commonly referred to as the kneecap, is the most recognised sesamoid bone, playing a crucial role in safeguarding the knee joint and enhancing the efficiency of muscle movement.

Osteogenesis and Maturation
The process of bone development initiates during the embryonic stage and persists into adulthood. Bones develop through two distinct processes: endochondral ossification (which facilitates the growth of long bones) and intramembranous ossification (responsible for the formation of flat bones, such as the skull). During the process of endochondral ossification, the cartilage structures that serve as precursors to bones are progressively substituted by bone tissue throughout an individual's growth.

Bone development persists throughout the stages of childhood and adolescence. The regions known as growth plates, found at the extremities of long bones, consist of cartilage that serves as the site for the generation of new bone cells. Upon reaching adulthood, the growth plates fuse, halting any further elongation of the bones.

Nonetheless, the process of replacing old bone with new bone, known as bone remodelling, persists throughout an individual's life. Osteoclasts, which are responsible for the resorption of bone, and osteoblasts, which facilitate the formation of new bone, collaborate to uphold bone integrity and facilitate repair processes.

Muscles: Function and Support

Categories of Muscular Tissue: Skeletal, Cardiac, and Smooth

Muscles are distinct types of tissues that generate force and facilitate movement. The human body comprises three varieties of muscle tissue, each serving unique roles:

1. Skeletal Muscle: These muscles connect to bones and facilitate voluntary movements, which are actions you can consciously regulate, including walking, running, and lifting objects. The appearance of skeletal muscles is characterised by a striated (striped) pattern, which results from the specific arrangement of muscle fibres. These muscles are typically connected to bones through tendons.

2. Cardiac Muscle: Exclusive to the heart, this type of muscle plays a crucial role in circulating blood throughout the body. In contrast to skeletal muscle, the contractions of cardiac muscle are involuntary, occurring without any conscious control. The muscle tissue of the heart exhibits striations and possesses the remarkable capacity to contract in a rhythmic and continuous manner without succumbing to fatigue.

3. Smooth Muscle: This muscle type is located in the walls of hollow organs, including the intestines, blood vessels, and bladder. Smooth muscle contractions occur without conscious control and lack striations. Smooth muscles play a crucial role in propelling food along the

digestive tract, adjusting the diameter of blood vessels, and managing bladder function.

The Mechanisms Behind Muscle Movement

Muscles operate through cycles of contraction and relaxation, facilitating movement. During muscle contraction, the muscle fibres shorten, exerting a pull on the attached bone, which results in the movement of that bone. Muscles function in pairs; as one muscle contracts (the agonist), the opposing muscle (the antagonist) relaxes. For instance, when you flex your elbow, the biceps muscle engages, while the triceps muscle releases. In the process of extending the elbow, the triceps engage while the biceps ease their tension.

Muscle contraction is initiated by electrical impulses originating from the nervous system. Upon the transmission of a signal from a motor neurone to a muscle fibre, there is a release of calcium ions within the muscle, which triggers a sequence of events leading to muscle contraction. When the signal ceases, the muscle undergoes relaxation.

Connective Tissues

Connective tissues such as tendons and ligaments are crucial components of the musculoskeletal system:
- Tendons: These structures serve to link muscles with bones. The force produced by muscle contraction is conveyed to the bone, facilitating movement. Tendons consist of resilient, fibrous tissue that is capable of enduring the significant forces generated during muscle activity.

- Ligaments: These structures serve to link bones together at joints, ensuring stability and limiting excessive motion. Ligaments consist of robust, fibrous tissue and are essential for maintaining joint stability during motion.

Articulations and Locomotion

Varieties of Articulations (Hinge, Ball and Socket, etc.) Joints serve as the connections between two or more bones, facilitating movement and providing flexibility. The specific joint structure dictates the extent and orientation of movement that can occur. The human body contains various types of joints:

1. Hinge Joints: These joints facilitate movement in a singular direction, akin to the mechanism of a door hinge. Instances of this phenomenon are seen in the elbow and knee, which facilitate flexion (bending) and extension (straightening).

2. Ball and Socket Joints: These joints feature a rounded bone end that fits into a cup-like socket, facilitating a broad spectrum of movement across various directions. The shoulder and hip joints function as ball and socket joints, allowing for movements such as rotation, abduction (moving away from the body), and adduction (moving towards the body).

3. Pivot Joints: These joints facilitate rotational movement around a singular axis. An illustration of this is the articulation between the initial two vertebrae, which facilitates the lateral rotation of the head.

4. Gliding Joints: These joints enable bones to smoothly slide past one another in any direction within the plane of the joint. Gliding joints are present in the wrists and ankles.

5. Saddle Joints: These joints facilitate movement across two dimensions, enabling both back-and-forth and side-to-side motion. The joint located at the base of the thumb serves as a prime illustration of a saddle joint.

6. Condyloid Joints: These joints facilitate movement while restricting rotation. These structures are located within the jaw and the joints of the fingers.

Function of Cartilage, Ligaments, and Synovial Fluid
A variety of elements collaborate to facilitate seamless and effective motion at the joints:

- Cartilage: This tissue is characterised by its smooth and flexible nature, serving to cover the ends of bones at joints. It plays a crucial role in minimising friction and acts as a cushion, preventing the bones from grinding against one another. Cartilage plays a crucial role in absorbing shock during movement.

- Ligaments: As previously stated, these structures serve to connect bones, providing stability to joints. They play a vital role in safeguarding against dislocation and limiting excessive movement that may harm the joint.

- Synovial Fluid: This viscous, lubricating substance is present within synovial joints, which facilitate movement, including those in the knee and elbow. This substance serves to lubricate the joint, minimising friction and wear on the cartilage. It additionally supports the cartilage by supplying it with essential nutrients.

The musculoskeletal system plays a crucial role in giving the body its framework, facilitating movement, and ensuring stability. The skeletal structure provides essential support for the organism, while muscular systems facilitate locomotion, and articulations enable diverse movements. Structures such as ligaments, tendons, cartilage, and synovial fluid are essential for maintaining efficient movement and protecting the body from injury. These elements function cohesively, enabling us to engage in everyday tasks, such as walking, running, lifting, and grasping items. Grasping the structure and function of the musculoskeletal system is essential for comprehending the mechanics of our bodies and their movements.

CHAPTER 4

The Nervous System

The nervous system constitutes an intricate web that governs and synchronises the various functions of the body. This system facilitates the exchange of information among various bodily components, enabling interaction with and reactions to our surroundings. The nervous system is categorised into two primary components: the central nervous system (CNS), encompassing the brain and spinal cord, and the peripheral nervous system (PNS), which comprises the nerves linking the CNS to the remainder of the body. This chapter delves into the intricate architecture and operations of the brain and spinal cord, examining the mechanisms of nerve communication, as well as the significance of reflexes and the autonomic nervous system in sustaining essential bodily functions.

The Central Nervous System: Command Centres

Central Nervous System: Brain and Spinal Cord
The central nervous system (CNS) serves as the body's command hub, tasked with processing information, making decisions, and orchestrating responses. The central nervous system consists of the brain and spinal cord, which collaborate to gather sensory information, interpret it, and relay commands to muscles and various tissues.

- The Brain: This organ is the most intricate in the human body, governing thought, memory, emotion, sensation, and movement. It has a mass of approximately three pounds and is segmented into distinct areas, each serving unique purposes.

- The Spinal Cord: The spinal cord is an elongated, slender assembly of nerve fibres that extends from the brain down through the vertebral column. This structure functions as a pathway for communication between the brain and the body, transmitting data from sensory receptors to the brain and directing motor instructions from the brain to the muscles. The spinal cord plays a crucial role in reflexes, serving as the pathway for automatic responses to various stimuli.

Roles of Various Areas of the Brain
The brain is organised into several key regions, each playing unique roles in regulating bodily functions:

1. Cerebrum: The cerebrum constitutes the most substantial segment of the brain, playing a crucial role in advanced cognitive processes including thought, reasoning, problem-solving, and decision-making. The structure is partitioned into two distinct hemispheres, each governing the functions of the opposite side of the body. The cerebrum is subdivided into four distinct lobes:
- Frontal Lobe: Plays a crucial role in voluntary movement, the production of speech, decision-making processes, and problem-solving abilities.
- Parietal Lobe: Engages in the processing of sensory data including touch, temperature, and pain sensations. It additionally contributes to understanding spatial relationships and navigating environments.
- Occipital Lobe: Plays a crucial role in interpreting visual stimuli received from the eyes.

- Temporal Lobe: Plays a crucial role in the processing of auditory stimuli and is vital for language comprehension and memory formation.

2. Cerebellum: Situated at the posterior aspect of the brain, the cerebellum is responsible for the coordination of muscle movements, the maintenance of posture, and the facilitation of balance. The cerebrum orchestrates voluntary movements, while the cerebellum fine-tunes them for smoothness and precision.

3. Brainstem: The brainstem serves as a crucial link between the brain and the spinal cord, regulating vital functions necessary for survival, including respiration, cardiac rhythm, and vascular pressure. It is composed of three primary components:
- Midbrain: Regulates reflexive responses associated with visual and auditory stimuli.
- Pons: Plays a crucial role in the regulation of breathing and acts as a vital communication link between the cerebrum and the cerebellum.
- Medulla Oblongata: Regulates essential involuntary processes including heartbeat, digestion, and the functioning of blood vessels.

The various areas of the brain collaborate seamlessly to interpret information, facilitate decision-making, and regulate both voluntary and involuntary movements.

Nerves: Pathways of Communication

Peripheral Nervous System: Sensory and Motor Nerves
The peripheral nervous system consists of all the nerves that branch out from the brain and spinal cord, reaching throughout the entire body. It serves as a vital conduit, relaying signals between the central nervous system

and different regions of the body. The peripheral nervous system can be classified into two primary categories:

- Sensory (Afferent) Nerves: These nerves transmit information from sensory receptors located in various parts of the body (including skin, eyes, and ears) to the central nervous system. These structures assist the brain and spinal cord in interpreting external stimuli, including touch, pain, temperature, sound, and light, enabling us to perceive and react to our surroundings.

- Motor (Efferent) Nerves: These nerves transmit signals from the central nervous system to muscles and glands, facilitating movement and action. Motor nerves can be classified into distinct categories:
- Somatic Motor Nerves: Regulate voluntary actions, including walking, lifting items, and verbal communication.
- Autonomic Motor Nerves: Regulate involuntary processes, including heartbeat, digestion, and glandular functions.

The Mechanisms Behind Movement and Sensory Perception

The nervous system orchestrates movement via a mechanism referred to as neuromuscular transmission. Upon the brain's decision to commence movement, motor neurones within the central nervous system transmit electrical impulses via motor nerves to the designated muscles. The release of calcium ions within the muscle cells is initiated by these signals, leading to contraction and the generation of movement. The integration of these signals facilitates seamless and regulated movements.

On the other hand, sensory nerves collect information from the environment and relay it to the central nervous system for processing. When you come into contact with a hot surface, sensory receptors in your skin transmit signals to your brain. The brain then interprets this sensation as pain and triggers a response to withdraw your hand.

Reflexes and Reaction

Basic Reflex Pathways and Their Significance
Reflexes are instinctive, unthinking reactions to particular stimuli that enable the body to respond swiftly to possible threats without requiring brain involvement. Reflex actions are governed by specific pathways known as reflex arcs, which engage solely the spinal cord and a limited number of neurones. This swift communication system guarantees that the organism can react nearly immediately to specific stimuli.

A straightforward reflex arc adheres to this fundamental pathway:
1. Stimulus: A sensory receptor identifies a stimulus, like the sensation of touching something hot.
2. Sensory Neurone: This type of neurone is responsible for conveying signals to the spinal cord.
3. Interneuron: Within the spinal cord, the sensory neurone forms a connection with an interneuron, which is responsible for processing the information.
4. Motor Neurone: The interneuron transmits a signal to a motor neurone, which conveys the command to a muscle or gland.
5. Response: The muscle contracts or the gland releases a substance, leading to a reflex action (e.g., withdrawing your hand from a hot surface).

Reflexes play a crucial role in safeguarding the body from injury while also ensuring stability and proper alignment. These reactions happen instinctively, enabling quick responses in scenarios that demand prompt action.

Autonomic Nervous System: Sympathetic vs. Parasympathetic
The autonomic nervous system (ANS) is a component of the peripheral nervous system responsible for controlling involuntary bodily functions, including heart rate, digestion, respiratory rate, and glandular activity. The autonomic nervous system consists of two branches that function in contrast to uphold homeostasis:

- Sympathetic Nervous System (SNS): The sympathetic nervous system is commonly known as the system that prepares the body for action in response to perceived threats. It primes the organism to react to stressful or perilous circumstances by elevating heart rate, widening air passages, and channelling blood flow towards the muscles. It also inhibits non-essential processes, like digestion, during periods of stress or crisis.

Essential roles of the sympathetic nervous system encompass: - Elevating heart rate and enhancing the strength of contractions.
- Expanding the pupils.
- Expanding air passages to enhance oxygen absorption.
- Diverting circulatory resources to the muscles involved in movement.
- Suppressing the functions of digestion and urination.

- Parasympathetic Nervous System (PNS): The parasympathetic nervous system is frequently referred to as the "rest and digest" system. It fosters a state of calm and recuperation by reducing the heart rate, enhancing digestive processes, and facilitating the removal of waste. The parasympathetic nervous system plays a crucial role in energy conservation and the regulation of routine physiological processes during periods of rest and relaxation.

Essential roles of the parasympathetic nervous system encompass: - Reducing the heart rate.
- Narrowing the pupils.
- Enhancing the processes of digestion and the secretion of saliva.
- Facilitating the process of bladder contraction and the expulsion of waste materials.

The sympathetic and parasympathetic systems collaborate intricately to manage physiological processes and uphold a state of balance within the body. For instance, following a stressful occurrence, the sympathetic system can elevate heart rate and enhance blood circulation to muscles, whereas the parasympathetic system subsequently aids in restoring the body to its typical resting condition.

The nervous system serves as the body's intricate control and communication network, enabling us to perceive our surroundings, make informed decisions, and react to various stimuli. The brain and spinal cord serve as the primary control hubs, with nerves facilitating the transmission of information across the body. Reflexes enable rapid, instinctive reactions to stimuli, while the autonomic nervous system oversees involuntary processes to sustain equilibrium and promote survival. Comprehending the architecture and role of the nervous system is crucial for appreciating how the body sustains its internal equilibrium and reacts to external stimuli.

CHAPTER 5

The Circulatory System

The circulatory system, often referred to as the cardiovascular system, plays a crucial role in sustaining life by facilitating the movement of nutrients, oxygen, hormones, and waste products throughout the organism. It is composed of three primary elements: the heart, the blood vessels, and the blood itself. The heart functions as the body's pump, while blood vessels serve as the conduits for circulation, and blood carries out essential roles in transport, defence, and regulation. This chapter delves into the intricate design and operation of the heart, the detailed anatomy of the circulatory system, and the essential role that blood serves in sustaining the body's physiological functions.

The Heart: The Organ of Circulation

Structure of the Heart: Compartments, Valvular System, and Circulatory Pathways
The heart is a muscular organ approximately the size of a fist, positioned slightly to the left of centre within the chest cavity. It functions as the essential pump of the circulatory system, driving blood circulation throughout the organism. The heart is composed of four distinct chambers along with essential valves and vessels that control the circulation of blood.

- Four Chambers: The heart consists of two upper sections known as atria and two lower sections referred to as ventricles. The atria are the chambers that accept

blood flowing into the heart, whereas the ventricles play a crucial role in ejecting blood from the heart.
- The right atrium collects deoxygenated blood from the body through the superior and inferior vena cavae.
- The left atrium takes in oxygen-rich blood from the lungs through the pulmonary veins.
- The right ventricle propels deoxygenated blood towards the lungs via the pulmonary artery for the purpose of oxygenation.
- The left ventricle is responsible for pumping oxygen-rich blood to the body via the aorta.
- Valves: The heart is equipped with four valves that regulate the flow of blood, ensuring it moves in the proper direction and preventing any backflow:
- The tricuspid valve is situated between the right atrium and the right ventricle.
- The pulmonary valve is located between the right ventricle and the pulmonary artery.
- The mitral valve is situated between the left atrium and the left ventricle.
- The aortic valve is located between the left ventricle and the aorta.

These valves operate rhythmically with each heartbeat, facilitating the seamless flow of blood through the heart and directing it into the appropriate vessels.

The Cardiac Cycle: Mechanisms of Blood Circulation
The rhythmic action of the heart is governed by a series of events known as the cardiac cycle, which unfolds with every heartbeat. The cycle consists of two primary phases: diastole and systole.

1. Diastole: In this phase, the heart muscles enter a state of relaxation, facilitating the filling of the atria with blood. As the chambers of the heart fill, pressure increases, leading to the opening of the tricuspid and

mitral valves. Blood subsequently enters the ventricles through passive flow.

2. Systole: This phase involves the contraction of the heart muscle. Upon reaching fullness, the ventricles contract, propelling blood into the pulmonary artery and aorta. The pulmonary valve facilitates the flow of blood into the lungs for oxygenation, whereas the aortic valve enables the distribution of oxygen-rich blood into the systemic circulation. At this stage, the atria initiate the process of refilling with blood in preparation for the subsequent cycle.

The complete cardiac cycle takes approximately 0.8 seconds in a healthy adult, facilitating the efficient pumping of blood throughout the body. The typical heart rate ranges from about 60 to 100 beats per minute, influenced by an individual's activity level.

Blood Vessels: Channels for Circulation

Categories of Blood Vessels: Arteries, Veins, Capillaries
The circulatory system consists of an intricate network of blood vessels that function as pathways for the movement of blood to and from the heart. Blood vessels can be classified into three primary categories:

- Arteries: These vessels transport oxygenated blood from the heart to the various tissues throughout the body. Arteries possess robust, muscular walls that enable them to endure the elevated pressure produced by the heart's rhythmic contractions. The aorta represents the most substantial artery within the organism, dividing into progressively smaller arteries and arterioles as it reaches the body's farthest points.

- Veins: These structures play a crucial role in transporting deoxygenated blood back to the heart. In contrast to arteries, veins possess walls that are less thick and include valves designed to inhibit the reverse flow of blood as it travels upward against gravity towards the heart. The superior and inferior vena cavae represent the largest veins in the circulatory system, transporting blood from the upper and lower regions of the body into the right atrium.

- Capillaries: These tiny blood vessels are the most abundant in the body, playing a crucial role in the circulatory system. These structures link arteries and veins, creating intricate networks that facilitate the transfer of oxygen, nutrients, and waste products between blood and tissues. The walls of capillaries are remarkably thin, facilitating the diffusion of gases, nutrients, and waste through their surfaces.

Haemodynamic Principles and Vascular Function
Hemodynamic pressure refers to the force that circulating fluid applies against the arterial walls throughout the organism. The two primary factors influencing this are the strength of the heart's contractions and the resistance encountered within the blood vessels. Blood pressure is generally assessed using two numerical values:
- Systolic pressure: The force exerted by circulating blood on the walls of the arteries during the contraction phase of the heart.
- Diastolic pressure: The pressure within the arteries during the relaxation phase of the cardiac cycle (diastole).

Maintaining proper circulation relies heavily on the importance of normal blood pressure. Elevated blood pressure can harm blood vessels and organs, whereas decreased blood pressure may lead to insufficient blood flow to essential organs.

The dynamics of circulation are influenced by peripheral resistance, which pertains to the opposition encountered by blood flow in the vessels. Arteries that exhibit enhanced elasticity and broader diameters facilitate smoother blood flow, whereas narrowed arteries can elevate resistance and lead to increased blood pressure.

Circulatory System: Transport and Immunity

Elements of Blood: Erythrocytes, Leukocytes, Thrombocytes, Serum
Blood is a unique bodily fluid that is essential for sustaining homeostasis. It consists of four primary elements:

1. Red Blood Cells (Erythrocytes): These cells play a crucial role in the transportation of oxygen from the lungs to various tissues, as well as facilitating the removal of carbon dioxide from the tissues back to the lungs for exhalation. These structures include haemoglobin, a crucial protein that attaches to oxygen, facilitating its distribution across the organism.

2. White Blood Cells (Leukocytes): These cells play a crucial role in the immune system, actively participating in the defence of the body against infections, diseases, and foreign invaders. Various categories of white blood cells exist, each fulfilling a distinct function in the immune system, such as neutrophils, lymphocytes, monocytes, eosinophils, and basophils.

3. Platelets (Thrombocytes): These tiny cell fragments are essential for the process of blood clotting. Upon

injury to a blood vessel, platelets gather at the location and secrete substances that trigger the clotting mechanism, aiding in the prevention of significant blood loss.

4. Plasma: Plasma constitutes the liquid component of blood, accounting for approximately 55% of its overall volume. The composition is mainly water, yet it also includes dissolved nutrients, hormones, electrolytes, and waste products. Plasma functions as a vital medium for the distribution of these substances throughout the body.

Roles of Blood in Oxygen Transport, Nutrient Distribution, and Immune Defence
Blood performs numerous critical roles that are fundamental for sustaining life:

1. Oxygen Transport: Red blood cells facilitate the movement of oxygen from the lungs to the tissues throughout the body. Haemoglobin found in red blood cells attaches to oxygen molecules, facilitating effective transport. After oxygen reaches the tissues, carbon dioxide, which is a byproduct of metabolic processes, is carried back to the lungs for exhalation.

2. Nutrient Delivery: The circulatory system transports vital nutrients, including glucose, amino acids, vitamins, and minerals, from the digestive tract to cells across the organism. These essential substances play a crucial role in generating energy, facilitating growth, and aiding in the repair of tissues.

3. Waste Removal: Blood gathers waste products, including urea and carbon dioxide, from the cells and carries them to the kidneys, liver, and lungs for elimination.

4. Immunity: The body's defenders, known as white blood cells, continuously navigate through the bloodstream and tissues, on the lookout for any indications of infection or damage. Upon the detection of a pathogen, such as bacteria or a virus, white blood cells spring into action, launching an immune response aimed at neutralising and eradicating the threat.

5. Blood Clotting: When a vessel is damaged, platelets and proteins in plasma collaborate to create blood clots, which help prevent excessive blood loss and support tissue repair.

The circulatory system is a complex web that guarantees the uninterrupted movement of blood across the entire body. The heart functions as the central pump, while blood vessels serve as the intricate pathways, and blood itself acts as the vital medium for the transportation of oxygen, nutrients, and immune cells throughout the body. Grasping the mechanics of this system is essential for preserving overall well-being and averting issues that impact circulation, including heart disease, hypertension, and anaemia.

CHAPTER 6

The Respiratory System

The respiratory system plays an essential role in the human body, facilitating the delivery of oxygen to the bloodstream while efficiently eliminating carbon dioxide, a byproduct of cellular respiration. This system is composed of the lungs, airways, and the muscles that facilitate respiration. This process enables the essential transfer of gases between the outside world and the circulatory system, guaranteeing that the organism receives sufficient oxygen for its operations while also allowing for the removal of carbon dioxide. This chapter explores the structure of the respiratory system, the processes involved in breathing, and the transportation of oxygen and carbon dioxide within the body.

Respiratory System: Facilitating Oxygen Intake

Structure of the Respiratory System: Nasal Cavities, Windpipe, Pulmonary Organs

The respiratory system is categorised into two main sections: the upper and lower respiratory tracts.

- Upper Respiratory Tract: The upper respiratory tract consists of the nasal passages, pharynx, and larynx.
- The nasal passages serve to filter, warm, and humidify the air we inhale. Microscopic hair-like formations known as cilia capture dust, pollen, and various foreign particles, effectively blocking their entry into the lungs.
- Air subsequently moves through the pharynx, also known as the throat, and the larynx, which is commonly

referred to as the voice box. The larynx houses the vocal cords, which oscillate to generate sound.

- Lower Respiratory Tract: The lower respiratory tract comprises the trachea, bronchi, bronchioles, and lungs.
- The trachea, commonly referred to as the windpipe, serves as a sturdy conduit for air, transporting it from the throat to the lungs. The structure is supported by C-shaped rings of cartilage that ensure it maintains its shape and does not collapse.
- The trachea divides into two bronchi, serving each lung individually. The bronchi continue to branch into smaller tubes known as bronchioles, culminating in groups of minute air sacs referred to as alveoli.

The Mechanism of Gas Exchange in Alveoli

The alveoli serve as the main locations for the exchange of gases within the lungs. These minute, balloon-shaped formations are enveloped by a web of capillaries, facilitating intimate interaction between air and blood. The alveolar walls possess remarkable thinness, enabling efficient gas exchange between the air within the alveoli and the blood in the adjacent capillaries.

- Gas Exchange: Upon inhalation, air abundant in oxygen enters the alveoli. Oxygen moves across the alveolar membrane into the bloodstream because of concentration differences, where it attaches to haemoglobin in red blood cells for distribution to various tissues in the body.

- Carbon Dioxide Removal: Concurrently, carbon dioxide, a byproduct of cellular metabolism, is transported by the bloodstream back to the lungs. Within the alveoli, carbon dioxide moves from the bloodstream into the air.

It is subsequently released from the organism during the process of exhalation.

The effectiveness of gas exchange is influenced by the surface area of the alveoli and the minimal thickness of the alveolar-capillary membrane. Conditions such as emphysema, characterised by damaged alveoli, or pulmonary fibrosis, which involves thickening and stiffening of lung tissue, can hinder this process.

Respiratory Processes

The Role of the Diaphragm and Intercostal Muscles in Breathing

Breathing is a mechanical process that consists of two phases: inhalation and exhalation. The phases are regulated by the contraction and relaxation of the diaphragm and intercostal muscles.

- Inhalation: During inhalation, the diaphragm, a dome-shaped muscle situated beneath the lungs, contracts and descends. Simultaneously, the muscles situated between the ribs contract, elevating the ribcage outward. This action enhances the capacity of the thoracic cavity, leading to a decrease in pressure within the lungs. Consequently, air enters the lungs to balance the pressure disparity between the interior and exterior of the body.

- Exhalation: The process of exhalation is generally considered to be passive. As the diaphragm and intercostal muscles relax, the volume of the chest cavity diminishes, leading to a rise in pressure within the lungs. This results in the expulsion of air from the lungs. During forced exhalation, like when engaging in intense physical activity or extinguishing candles, the internal intercostal muscles contract to decrease the thoracic cavity's volume, allowing for a more powerful expulsion of air.

Control of Respiration by the Central Nervous System

The rate and depth of breathing are controlled by the respiratory centres located in the brainstem, particularly within the medulla oblongata and the pons. These centres react to alterations in the chemical composition of the blood, including fluctuations in oxygen, carbon dioxide, and hydrogen ion concentrations (pH).

- Chemoreceptors located in the brain and blood vessels are responsible for detecting the levels of carbon dioxide and pH in the bloodstream. As carbon dioxide concentrations increase, the acidity of the blood elevates, resulting in a decreased pH level. In response, the medulla oblongata transmits signals to enhance both the rate and depth of respiration, facilitating the expulsion of greater amounts of carbon dioxide and aiding in the restoration of normal pH levels.

- Likewise, when oxygen levels drop significantly, the brain prompts an elevation in the breathing rate to enhance the intake of oxygen into the lungs.

This feedback mechanism guarantees that respiration adapts in response to the body's metabolic requirements, whether during physical activity or periods of rest.

Transport of Oxygen and Carbon Dioxide

The Mechanism of Oxygen Transport in Blood

After oxygen enters the bloodstream in the lungs, it is essential for it to be delivered to various cells across the body to facilitate the process of cellular respiration. Oxygen is mainly transported in the bloodstream by haemoglobin, a protein located in red blood cells.

- Each haemoglobin molecule has the capacity to bind with four oxygen molecules. In the lungs, where oxygen concentration is elevated, haemoglobin attaches to oxygen and creates oxyhemoglobin. As blood flows through the body and encounters areas with diminished oxygen concentrations, haemoglobin discharges the oxygen, allowing it to permeate into the cells.

- A minor fraction of oxygen is also found dissolved directly in the blood plasma, yet this represents only a small part of the overall oxygen transport process.

The capacity of haemoglobin to attach to and release oxygen is affected by various elements, such as temperature, pH, and carbon dioxide concentrations. In active tissues characterised by elevated carbon dioxide levels and reduced pH (more acidic conditions), haemoglobin exhibits a greater tendency to release oxygen—this is referred to as the Bohr effect. This guarantees that oxygen reaches the areas that require it the most, particularly in active muscles during physical activity.

Elimination of Carbon Dioxide

Carbon dioxide (CO_2) is a byproduct produced during the process of cellular respiration. Once cells utilise oxygen to generate energy, they produce carbon dioxide as a byproduct, which needs to be expelled from the body to avoid detrimental accumulation.

Carbon dioxide is carried from the tissues to the lungs through three primary mechanisms:

1. Dissolved in Plasma: A minor fraction of carbon dioxide (approximately 5-7%) is directly dissolved in the blood plasma.

2. Bicarbonate Ions: The majority of carbon dioxide (about 70%) is transformed into bicarbonate ions (HCO_3^-) within the bloodstream. This reaction is facilitated by the enzyme carbonic anhydrase found in red blood cells. During this process, carbon dioxide interacts with water to produce carbonic acid (H_2CO_3), which rapidly breaks down into bicarbonate ions and hydrogen ions. The bicarbonate ions are subsequently carried in the plasma to the lungs, where the reaction is reversed, allowing carbon dioxide to be expelled during exhalation.

3. Carbaminohemoglobin: Approximately 20-25% of carbon dioxide attaches to haemoglobin, resulting in the formation of carbaminohemoglobin. In contrast to oxygen, which attaches to the iron found in haemoglobin, carbon dioxide interacts with the protein component of haemoglobin. As blood flows into the lungs, carbon dioxide is released from haemoglobin and diffuses into the alveoli, where it is expelled from the body.

Sustaining pH Equilibrium

The movement of carbon dioxide is crucial for sustaining the pH equilibrium of the blood. The transformation of carbon dioxide into bicarbonate ions functions as a buffering mechanism that aids in maintaining the acidity levels of the blood. When there is an elevation in carbon dioxide levels leading to heightened acidity, the respiratory system responds by accelerating the breathing rate to eliminate surplus carbon dioxide and re-establish pH equilibrium.

The respiratory system collaborates closely with the circulatory system to ensure that oxygen reaches the body's cells while facilitating the removal of carbon dioxide. The lungs, airways, and muscles involved in breathing form a complex system for gas exchange, with the brain regulating the process to align with the body's requirements. Comprehending the role of the respiratory system is crucial for recognising how the body sustains balance and adapts to different needs and environmental shifts.

CHAPTER 7

The Digestive System

The digestive system plays a crucial role in transforming the food we ingest into vital nutrients that our bodies utilise for energy, growth, and the repair of cells. This intricate system comprises various organs and processes that collaborate to decompose food, assimilate nutrients, and expel waste. Comprehending the intricacies of the digestive system is essential for grasping the influence of our dietary selections on our overall well-being. This chapter will delve into the intricacies of the digestive process, examining how nutrients are absorbed and the functions of digestive enzymes and hormones.

Examination of the Digestive Process

The Process of Digestion and Nutrient Absorption

The process of digestion initiates the moment food is introduced into the oral cavity. The process of food travelling through the digestive system consists of distinct phases: ingestion, digestion, absorption, and elimination.

1. Ingestion: Ingestion refers to the process of consuming food via the oral cavity. This process is enhanced by chewing, where the teeth fragment food into smaller pieces, thereby increasing the surface area for enzymes to interact with. Saliva, generated by the salivary glands, is rich in enzymes like amylase, initiating the process of carbohydrate breakdown.

2. Digestion: This process encompasses both mechanical and chemical breakdown of food:
- Physical Breakdown of Food: This process takes place via the mechanical breakdown of food through mastication and the rhythmic contractions of the stomach. The muscles of the stomach work to blend food with gastric juices, transforming it into a semi-liquid substance known as chyme.
- Chemical Breakdown: Enzymatic processes decompose macromolecules into their fundamental components. Carbohydrates break down into simple sugars, proteins decompose into amino acids, and fats are converted into fatty acids and glycerol. The process of chemical digestion persists within the stomach and small intestine.

3. Absorption: Following the process of digestion, nutrients are taken up by the body through the intestinal walls. The small intestine serves as the main location for nutrient absorption, facilitating the transfer of nutrients through the intestinal lining into the bloodstream.

4. Elimination: Ultimately, any undigested food and waste products are expelled from the body through the large intestine and released via the rectum.

Components of the Digestive System: Oral Cavity, Oesophagus, Gastric Chamber, Intestinal Tract

The primary organs engaged in the process of digestion consist of:

- Mouth: The initial site for food intake, where the process of mechanical breakdown commences through chewing, and the onset of chemical breakdown occurs with saliva.

- Oesophagus: A dynamic conduit that links the oral cavity to the stomach. The act of swallowing propels food into the oesophagus, where a series of rhythmic contractions known as peristalsis transport it towards the stomach.

- Stomach: A robust organ that combines food with gastric secretions, which include hydrochloric acid and digestive enzymes. The acidic environment facilitates the breakdown of proteins and eliminates harmful bacteria.

- Small Intestine: Consisting of three distinct sections (duodenum, jejunum, and ileum), this organ is the primary site for digestion and the absorption of nutrients. Digestive enzymes produced by the pancreas and bile secreted by the liver play a crucial role in the further breakdown of food.

- Large Intestine: Commonly referred to as the colon, this organ plays a crucial role in absorbing water and electrolytes, while also forming and storing waste prior to its elimination. It also contains advantageous microorganisms that assist in the digestive process.

Uptake of Nutrients

Role of the Small Intestine in Nutrient Uptake

The small intestine serves as the primary location for the absorption of most nutrients. The design is finely tuned for this purpose, incorporating various characteristics:

- Villi and Microvilli: The inner lining of the small intestine features numerous minute, finger-like projections known as villi. Each villus is further lined with even smaller projections known as microvilli, which greatly enhance the surface area. This large surface area facilitates a more effective uptake of nutrients.

- Nutrient Transport: Nutrients that are absorbed via the intestinal walls make their way into the bloodstream or lymphatic system. Simple sugars and amino acids enter the bloodstream directly, whereas fatty acids and glycerol are taken up by the lymphatic system.

- Targeted Transport Processes: Various nutrients necessitate distinct transport processes for optimal absorption. For instance, certain nutrients enter cells through passive diffusion, whereas others necessitate active transport or facilitated diffusion, which relies on carrier proteins.

The small intestine plays a crucial role in efficiently absorbing nutrients, which is vital for supplying the body with the energy and building blocks needed for numerous physiological processes.

Function of the Large Intestine in Maintaining Hydration and Waste Production

The large intestine is essential for regulating the body's water balance and for the formation of waste products that are ready for elimination. The roles it plays encompass:

- Water Absorption: As the semi-fluid mixture progresses into the large intestine, it predominantly consists of liquid. The large intestine plays a crucial role in absorbing water and electrolytes, converting the liquid chyme into a more solid state. This mechanism is crucial for sustaining hydration and ensuring the proper balance of electrolytes within the organism.

- Formation of Faeces: The leftover undigested substances, in conjunction with metabolic waste, undergo compaction into faeces as water is absorbed. The large intestine serves as a habitat for advantageous microorganisms that break down undigested carbohydrates, generating short-chain fatty acids that the body can absorb and use effectively.

- Storage and Elimination: The large intestine serves as a reservoir for faecal matter until it is time for it to be expelled from the body via the rectum. The process of elimination is referred to as defecation, governed by the autonomic nervous system and encompassing both involuntary and voluntary muscle contractions.

Enzymes and Hormonal Regulation of Digestion

Significance of Catalysts in Food Decomposition

Digestive enzymes serve as catalysts that aid in the decomposition of food into its essential nutrients. They play an essential role in the digestive process and are generated in different regions of the digestive system:

- Salivary Amylase: This enzyme, generated in the salivary glands, initiates the process of carbohydrate digestion right in the mouth.

- Pepsin: Produced by the stomach lining, pepsin is an enzyme responsible for breaking down proteins into smaller peptides. It becomes active in the acidic conditions found within the stomach.

- Pancreatic Enzymes: The pancreas generates a variety of crucial enzymes that are secreted into the small intestine:
- Pancreatic Amylase: Plays a crucial role in the ongoing process of carbohydrate digestion.
- Trypsin and Chymotrypsin: Catalyse the hydrolysis of proteins, resulting in the formation of smaller peptide fragments.
- Lipase: Breaks down fats into fatty acids and glycerol.

- Intestinal Enzymes: The cells that line the small intestine produce more enzymes, such as maltase, lactase, and sucrase, which continue the process of breaking down disaccharides into monosaccharides.

These enzymes function best at particular pH levels and temperatures, guaranteeing that food is effectively decomposed for nutrient uptake.

The Role of Hormones in Digestive Regulation

Hormones are essential in managing the digestive process, orchestrating the functions of different organs that contribute to digestion. Essential hormones consist of:

- Gastrin: This hormone is synthesised in the stomach when food is consumed, prompting the release of gastric juices such as hydrochloric acid and pepsinogen, which play a crucial role in protein digestion.

- Secretin: When acidic chyme from the stomach enters the small intestine, this hormone is released to prompt the pancreas to secrete bicarbonate. This process neutralises stomach acid, creating an ideal pH environment for the functioning of intestinal enzymes.

- Cholecystokinin (CCK): This peptide hormone is secreted by the small intestine when it detects the presence of fatty acids and amino acids. Its primary functions include stimulating the gallbladder to release bile, which is essential for fat digestion, and enhancing the secretion of pancreatic enzymes.

- Ghrelin and Leptin: These hormones play crucial roles in managing appetite and the feeling of fullness, respectively. Ghrelin plays a crucial role in enhancing appetite, whereas leptin serves as a signal for satiety, contributing to the regulation of food consumption.

The interaction of these hormones guarantees that the digestive system reacts suitably to food consumption, enhancing digestion and nutrient uptake.

The digestive system represents an intricate and essential framework that converts food into crucial nutrients while also expelling waste products. Grasping the mechanisms of digestion, absorption, and the functions of enzymes and hormones is essential for recognising how the body sustains itself and upholds health. A properly operating digestive system is crucial for maintaining overall health, and any disturbances in this system can result in a range of health problems. By acknowledging the significance of healthy eating patterns and comprehending the mechanisms through which our bodies metabolise food, we can make educated decisions that enhance our digestive wellness and overall health.

CHAPTER 8

The Urinary System

The urinary system is essential for sustaining the body's internal environment, as it filters waste products from the blood, regulates fluid and electrolyte balance, and manages blood pressure. This system consists of multiple organs that collaborate to efficiently remove waste, safeguard vital nutrients, and uphold a balanced internal environment. This chapter delves into the structure and role of the kidneys, the process of urine formation, and the mechanisms involved in blood pressure regulation.

Kidneys: The Body's Blood Purifiers

Structure and Role of the Kidneys

The kidneys are paired, bean-shaped structures situated in the lower back, flanking the spine on either side. The dimensions of each kidney range from about 4 to 5 inches in length, featuring a sophisticated internal architecture that enables it to carry out essential functions with great efficiency.

1. Structure of the Kidneys: - Cortex and Medulla: The outer layer of the kidney is referred to as the cortex, whereas the inner region is identified as the medulla. The cortex houses nephrons, which serve as the kidney's functional units, whereas the medulla consists of renal pyramids that facilitate urine collection and drainage.
- Nephrons: Each kidney is home to approximately a million nephrons, the tiny structures that play a crucial

role in filtering blood and generating urine. Each nephron is composed of a glomerulus, which is a network of capillaries, and a renal tubule, a series of tubules that alter the filtrate.
- Pelvis and Ureter: The central region of the kidney is referred to as the renal pelvis, which gathers urine produced by the nephrons and channels it into the ureter, a conduit that carries urine to the bladder.

2. Functions of the Kidneys: - Filtration: The main role of the kidneys is to remove waste products and surplus substances from the bloodstream. This process of filtration takes place in the glomeruli, where the pressure of blood drives fluid and small solutes through the walls of the capillaries into the renal tubules.
- Reabsorption: Following the filtration process, the renal tubules reclaim crucial nutrients, electrolytes, and water, returning them to the bloodstream to maintain the retention of essential substances.
- Secretion: The kidneys play a crucial role in the elimination of waste products and surplus ions by secreting them into the tubules for excretion, thereby preserving the body's substance equilibrium.
- Excretion: The end result, urine, consists of waste materials and surplus substances that are eliminated from the body.

The Role of Kidneys in Regulating Fluid and Electrolyte Homeostasis

The kidneys are essential for maintaining the balance of fluids and electrolytes in the body. They accomplish this using a range of mechanisms:

1. Fluid Balance: The kidneys regulate urine production in response to the body's hydration levels. When fluid intake increases, the kidneys respond by excreting a

greater volume of urine to remove surplus water from the body. On the other hand, when there is insufficient fluid intake, the kidneys adapt by conserving water, leading to more concentrated urine and a decrease in urine volume.

2. Electrolyte Regulation: The kidneys maintain the balance of essential electrolytes, including sodium, potassium, calcium, and chloride. They accomplish this through:
- Reabsorption: The renal tubules selectively reclaim electrolytes, returning them to the bloodstream according to the body's requirements.
- Secretion: The kidneys have the ability to release surplus electrolytes into the urine for elimination.

3. Acid-Base Balance: The kidneys contribute to the maintenance of the body's acid-base equilibrium by excreting hydrogen ions and reabsorbing bicarbonate ions, thereby regulating blood pH.

The kidneys play a crucial role in maintaining balance by effectively managing fluid and electrolyte levels, which is essential for the smooth operation of bodily functions.

The Process of Urine Formation

Mechanism of Blood Filtration and Urine Production

The formation of urine takes place through three primary stages: filtration, reabsorption, and secretion.

1. Filtration: - Blood flows into the kidneys via the renal arteries, which divide into smaller arterioles and eventually reach the glomeruli. In this process, the pressure inside the capillaries drives water, electrolytes, and small molecules like glucose and amino acids into

the Bowman's capsule, resulting in the formation of glomerular filtrate.
- Typically, larger molecules like proteins and blood cells are too substantial to traverse the filtration barrier, thus remaining within the bloodstream.

2. Reabsorption: - Following filtration, the glomerular filtrate moves through the renal tubules (proximal convoluted tubule, loop of Henle, distal convoluted tubule), where the process of reabsorption takes place.
- Within the proximal convoluted tubule, a considerable quantity of water, glucose, and sodium ions is reabsorbed into the bloodstream. The loop of Henle plays a crucial role in urine concentration through the reabsorption of water and sodium, enhancing the body's ability to manage fluid balance. In the distal convoluted tubule and collecting duct, further reabsorption takes place according to the body's requirements.

3. Secretion: - The renal tubules play a crucial role in eliminating extra waste products, including hydrogen ions, creatinine, and specific medications, into the tubular fluid. This mechanism plays a crucial role in maintaining the blood's composition and facilitating the removal of waste products.

4. Urine Formation: - The end result, urine, is created as the leftover fluid moves through the collecting ducts, where it undergoes concentration. Urine consists of a mixture of water, urea, creatinine, uric acid, electrolytes, and a range of waste products.

Function of the Bladder and Urethra in Waste Elimination

After urine is produced, it travels from the kidneys to the urinary bladder through the ureters.

1. Bladder: - The bladder functions as a muscular sac, acting as a temporary storage reservoir for urine. The structure is capable of both expansion and contraction as it undergoes the processes of filling and emptying, enabling the organism to regulate the timing of urination effectively. The walls of the bladder are composed of smooth muscle fibres that contract to aid in the expulsion of urine.

2. Urethra: - The urethra serves as a conduit, linking the bladder to the external environment. In males, the structure is elongated and fulfils two roles (urinary and reproductive), whereas in females, it is more compact and exclusively serves the urinary purpose. The act of excretion, commonly known as urination, takes place when the bladder contracts, propelling urine into the urethra, from where it is released from the body through the voluntary control of the external urethral sphincter.

Control of Blood Pressure

The Role of Kidneys in Blood Pressure and Volume Regulation

The kidneys are essential in maintaining blood pressure, utilising various mechanisms, with a key focus on the renin-angiotensin-aldosterone system (RAAS).

1. Renin Release: - When blood pressure decreases or there is a reduction in sodium chloride concentration within the nephron, specialised cells in the kidneys known as juxtaglomerular cells release the enzyme renin into the bloodstream. This enzyme triggers a

series of reactions that eventually result in the formation of angiotensin II.

2. Angiotensin II: - Angiotensin II serves as a powerful agent that constricts blood vessels, thereby elevating blood pressure. This process also activates the adrenal glands to secrete aldosterone, a hormone that facilitates the reabsorption of sodium and water in the kidneys, resulting in an increase in blood volume and a subsequent rise in blood pressure.

3. Antidiuretic Hormone (ADH): - The kidneys react to signals from ADH, a hormone secreted by the pituitary gland in response to dehydration in the body. ADH enhances the permeability of the renal collecting ducts, facilitating greater water reabsorption into the bloodstream, which in turn elevates blood volume and pressure.

4. Natriuresis: - The kidneys play a crucial role in maintaining blood pressure by eliminating surplus sodium and water, a mechanism referred to as natriuresis. The elimination of sodium results in a reduction of blood volume, which subsequently leads to a decrease in blood pressure.

5. Feedback Mechanisms: - The kidneys play a crucial role in regulating blood pressure and volume by utilising specialised cells that constantly assess these parameters, making necessary adjustments to ensure balance within the body. As blood pressure increases, the kidneys can lower the secretion of renin, which results in a reduction of both blood volume and pressure.

The urinary system plays a crucial role in filtering waste products from the bloodstream, ensuring fluid and electrolyte balance, and regulating blood pressure. The kidneys, serving as the main organs of this system, execute intricate functions that help maintain the body's equilibrium. By exploring the structure and function of the urinary system, we can acknowledge its crucial contribution to overall health and understand the significance of preserving kidney function through adequate hydration, a nutritious diet, and sound lifestyle practices.

CHAPTER 9

The Endocrine System

The endocrine system comprises a sophisticated array of glands and hormones that oversee a variety of essential bodily functions, such as metabolism, growth, development, and reproduction. It serves an essential function in preserving equilibrium—the condition of stability within the organism. This chapter delves into the definition and function of hormones, the primary endocrine glands, and the significance of hormonal regulation in maintaining homeostasis, particularly emphasising insulin and its role in blood sugar regulation.

Hormones: Essential Chemical Signals

Understanding the Function and Impact of Hormones on Bodily Processes

Hormones are intricate biochemical substances synthesised by a variety of glands within the endocrine system. These substances function as signalling molecules that move through the circulatory system to specific organs and tissues, where they produce their effects. Hormones play a crucial role in regulating numerous physiological processes, such as:

1. Metabolism: Hormones play a crucial role in regulating metabolic pathways, affecting the body's utilisation of energy and nutrients. Insulin is essential for the process of glucose metabolism.

2. Growth and Development: Hormones like growth hormone (GH) play a crucial role in promoting growth and development throughout childhood and adolescence, influencing factors such as bone length, muscle mass, and overall body composition.

3. Reproductive Functions: Hormones like oestrogen and testosterone play essential roles in sexual development and the processes of reproduction. They control the menstrual cycle, the production of sperm, and the development of secondary sexual traits.

4. Response to Stress: Hormones such as cortisol, generated by the adrenal glands, facilitate the body's reaction to stress by elevating blood sugar levels and modifying metabolism.

5. Homeostasis: Hormones play a crucial role in sustaining the internal environment of the body by overseeing functions like blood pressure, fluid balance, and electrolyte levels.

Primary Hormonal Structures

The system of glands responsible for hormone production and secretion includes several essential components:

1. Pituitary Gland: Commonly known as the master gland, this structure is situated at the base of the brain and oversees the activities of other endocrine glands. This organ synthesises various hormones, including growth hormone, prolactin, and adrenocorticotropic hormone (ACTH).

2. Thyroid Gland: Situated in the neck, this gland synthesises hormones (T3 and T4) that play a crucial

role in regulating metabolism, energy production, and the overall growth and development of the organism. It additionally produces calcitonin, a hormone that plays a crucial role in maintaining calcium balance in the bloodstream.

3. Adrenal Glands: Located on top of each kidney, these glands are responsible for the production of hormones like cortisol (which plays a role in the stress response), aldosterone (which helps regulate sodium and potassium levels), and adrenaline (epinephrine, which readies the body for fight-or-flight reactions).

4. Pancreas: This organ operates in dual capacities, serving as both an endocrine and exocrine gland. In its role within the endocrine system, it synthesises insulin and glucagon, which are crucial hormones for the regulation of blood sugar levels.

5. Gonads: The ovaries and testes are crucial for the production of sex hormones, such as oestrogen, progesterone, and testosterone, which are essential for reproductive functions and the development of secondary sexual characteristics.

6. Pineal Gland: This gland is responsible for the production of melatonin, a hormone that plays a crucial role in regulating sleep-wake cycles and circadian rhythms.

7. Thymus: Found in the upper chest, this organ is responsible for producing thymosin, a hormone crucial for the development of the immune system, especially in childhood.

Each of these glands plays a vital role in the complex system of hormonal communication that governs numerous physiological processes.

Balance and Hormonal Control

The Role of Hormones in Regulating Growth, Metabolism, and Reproductive Processes

The endocrine system is crucial for sustaining homeostasis, as it regulates numerous physiological processes via hormonal signalling. Hormonal regulation encompasses complex feedback systems that guarantee the body operates at its best.

1. Growth Regulation: Hormones like growth hormone and thyroid hormones collaborate to control growth and development. Growth hormone facilitates the development of bones and tissues, whereas thyroid hormones play a crucial role in regulating metabolic rates, ensuring that energy is accessible for growth activities.

2. Metabolic Regulation: Hormones play a vital role in the regulation of metabolism, encompassing the breakdown of carbohydrates, proteins, and fats. Insulin and glucagon, both secreted by the pancreas, function in opposition to regulate blood glucose concentrations within a precise range. Insulin aids in the absorption of glucose by cells, encouraging its utilisation for energy or its storage as glycogen, whereas glucagon initiates the release of glucose from stored glycogen when blood sugar levels decrease.

3. Reproductive Regulation: Hormones play a crucial role in controlling the menstrual cycle in females and the process of spermatogenesis in males. For example,

oestrogen and progesterone play crucial roles in managing the menstrual cycle, whereas testosterone is vital for the production of sperm and the emergence of male secondary sexual traits. Hormonal imbalances can result in reproductive challenges, underscoring the significance of effective hormonal regulation.

4. Stress Response: Hormones like cortisol are secreted when faced with stress, leading to physiological alterations such as elevated blood sugar levels and improved energy accessibility. This reaction is essential for endurance, enabling the organism to manage pressing dangers.

Illustration: Insulin and the Control of Blood Glucose Levels

A prominent illustration of hormonal control is the function of insulin in managing blood sugar levels:

1. Insulin Production: The beta cells of the pancreas synthesise insulin when blood glucose levels rise, particularly following a meal. Upon the digestion of carbohydrates, glucose is absorbed into the bloodstream, prompting the pancreas to secrete insulin.

2. Mechanism of Action: Insulin promotes the absorption of glucose by specific cells, especially within muscle and adipose (fat) tissues. This process facilitates the transformation of glucose into glycogen, allowing for its storage in the liver and muscles. Furthermore, insulin acts to suppress gluconeogenesis, which is the mechanism of generating glucose from sources other than carbohydrates, thereby contributing to a reduction in blood sugar levels.

3. Preserving Internal Balance: Insulin is essential for facilitating the uptake and storage of glucose, thereby playing a vital role in the prevention of hyperglycemia and the maintenance of energy equilibrium. As blood sugar levels decrease, the pancreas diminishes its release of insulin, facilitating the stabilisation of glucose levels.

4. Diabetes and Hormonal Imbalance: In those affected by diabetes, the production or action of insulin is compromised, resulting in persistently elevated blood sugar levels. Type 1 diabetes arises from the immune system's attack on beta cells, resulting in inadequate insulin production. Type 2 diabetes is characterised by insulin resistance, a condition in which cells fail to respond adequately to insulin. Both conditions can lead to significant health issues if not addressed appropriately.

5. Feedback Mechanisms: The control of blood sugar operates through a negative feedback loop. When glucose concentrations increase, insulin is secreted to bring them down. On the other hand, when blood sugar levels decrease, glucagon is released to elevate them, maintaining glucose levels within a healthy range.

The endocrine system plays a crucial role in managing various bodily functions by releasing hormones. These chemical signals regulate internal balance by overseeing growth, metabolism, reproduction, and reactions to stress. By exploring the functions of different hormones and the processes they engage in, we can recognise the intricate equilibrium that maintains the body's optimal performance. The case of insulin and its role in regulating blood sugar underscores the vital significance of hormonal balance in preserving overall well-being.

CHAPTER 10

The Immune System

The immune system serves as the body's protective barrier, meticulously crafted to shield against detrimental pathogens, including bacteria, viruses, and fungi. It serves a vital function in sustaining well-being and averting illnesses. This chapter will delve into the functions of the immune system, the various types of immunity, the organs that play a role in immune responses, and the significance of vaccines in developing and strengthening immunity.

The Body's Protective System

Examination of the Immune System's Function in Defending Against Pathogens

The immune system comprises a sophisticated array of cells, tissues, and organs that collaborate to protect the body from harmful intruders. The main roles encompass recognising harmful microorganisms, counteracting their effects, and removing them from the organism. The immune response is primarily divided into two fundamental categories: innate immunity and adaptive immunity.

- Innate Immunity: This represents the body's initial protective mechanism, encompassing physical barriers like skin and mucous membranes, along with immune cells that react swiftly to invading pathogens. Innate immunity operates in a non-specific manner, indicating that it does not focus on particular pathogens but instead reacts to a broad array of possible dangers.

Elements of the body's natural defence system consist of:

- Physical Barriers: The skin, mucous membranes, and secretions such as tears and saliva serve as protective barriers to inhibit the entry of pathogens.

- Cellular Defences: White blood cells, including phagocytes and natural killer cells, are crucial in identifying and eliminating pathogens.

- Inflammatory Response: Upon injury or infection of tissues, a response is triggered that results in heightened blood flow, swelling, and the mobilisation of immune cells to the affected area.

- Adaptive Immunity: This response is tailored and evolves as the organism interacts with various pathogens over time. Adaptive immunity is defined by its capacity to recall past infections, facilitating a quicker and more efficient reaction when encountering the same pathogen again. Essential characteristics consist of:

- Lymphocytes: The two primary types of lymphocytes, B cells and T cells, play essential roles in the adaptive immune response. B cells generate antibodies aimed at particular pathogens, whereas T cells play a crucial role in modulating the immune response and directly eliminating infected cells.

- Immunological Memory: Following an infection, memory B cells and memory T cells persist in the body, facilitating a quicker and stronger immune response upon re-exposure to the pathogen.

Components of the Immune System

Lymphatic Structures, Immune Organ, Endocrine Gland, and Haematopoietic Tissue

The immune system consists of a diverse array of organs and tissues that play crucial roles in its functions. These consist of:

1. Bone Marrow: This tissue serves as the main location for the generation of blood cells, encompassing red blood cells, white blood cells, and platelets. This is the site where haematopoietic stem cells undergo differentiation into diverse immune cell types, such as B cells and other lymphocytes.

2. Thymus: This organ is uniquely positioned behind the sternum, playing a crucial role in the immune system. The maturation of T cells is crucial, as these cells are fundamental to the adaptive immune response. In the early stages of life, T cells travel from the bone marrow to the thymus, where they undergo maturation and develop the ability to differentiate between the body's own cells and external threats.

3. Lymph Nodes: These are small, bean-shaped structures that are found throughout the body. These structures function as essential filters for lymph fluid, capturing pathogens and debris effectively. Lymph nodes house a significant population of immune cells, especially B and T cells, which can be triggered upon the detection of pathogens. Enlarged lymph nodes frequently signify a vigorous immune reaction to an infection.

4. Spleen: This organ is the largest within the lymphatic system and is situated in the upper left region of the

abdomen. This organ plays a crucial role in purifying blood by eliminating aged or impaired red blood cells, harmful pathogens, and cellular waste. The spleen houses immune cells capable of reacting to pathogens present in the bloodstream, playing a crucial role in the body's defence systems.

5. Mucosal Associated Lymphoid Tissue (MALT): This encompasses structures such as the tonsils and Peyer's patches found within the intestines. MALT is essential for safeguarding mucosal surfaces and blocking the entry of pathogens.

Function of Immune Cells in Combatting Infections

Leukocytes play a vital role in the immune system, tasked with the identification and eradication of pathogens. These can be categorised into various types, such as:

1. Phagocytes: This group comprises neutrophils and macrophages, which capture and break down pathogens via a mechanism known as phagocytosis.
2. Lymphocytes: As noted earlier, B cells generate antibodies that attach to particular pathogens, signalling them for elimination. T cells play a crucial role in directly eliminating infected cells and modulating the immune response through signalling to other immune components.

3. Natural Killer Cells: These cells are essential for identifying and eliminating infected or malignant cells without needing previous exposure to the pathogen.

4. Dendritic Cells: These specialised cells play a crucial role in capturing and processing antigens, subsequently

presenting them to T cells to kickstart the adaptive immune response.

Vaccines and Immune Response

Understanding the Mechanism of Vaccines in Immune System Training

Vaccination stands out as a highly effective approach in safeguarding public health against infectious diseases. Vaccines function by activating the immune system to identify and retain memory of particular pathogens while preventing the onset of the disease itself. The procedure encompasses multiple essential stages:

1. Introduction of Antigens: Vaccines consist of attenuated or inactivated components of a pathogen, including proteins or sugars that act as antigens. These antigens elicit a response from the immune system.

2. Initiation of the Immune Response: Upon the administration of a vaccine, the immune system identifies the antigens as non-self entities. B cells generate antibodies, while T cells become activated to identify and eliminate infected cells.

3. Formation of Immunological Memory: Following the immune response, memory B cells and memory T cells are generated. These cells persist within the organism, contributing to enduring immunity.

4. Swift Reaction to Future Pathogen Exposure: Should the vaccinated person come into contact with the genuine pathogen later on, the immune system is capable of launching a rapid and efficient defence, averting disease.

Significance of Immune Function in Well-being

1. Disease Prevention: Vaccines have significantly reduced the prevalence of numerous infectious diseases, including smallpox and polio, approaching their elimination. They safeguard not just those who have received vaccinations but also play a crucial role in fostering herd immunity, thereby offering protection to individuals who are unable to be vaccinated for medical reasons.

2. Mitigation of Disease Impact: Individuals who have received vaccinations and still contract the illness typically exhibit less severe symptoms than those who are unvaccinated, leading to fewer hospital admissions and lower healthcare expenses.

3. Public Health: The implementation of widespread vaccination is essential for managing outbreaks and halting the transmission of infectious diseases among populations. It plays a vital role in enhancing the overall health and well-being of the population.

4. Evolving Threats: With the emergence of new pathogens, the capacity to adapt and create innovative vaccines is crucial for safeguarding public health. Ongoing exploration and innovation in the field of immunology and vaccine technology are essential for the fight against diseases.

5. Global Health Initiatives: Vaccination programs play a crucial role in global health initiatives, especially in regions with limited access to healthcare resources. Vaccines play a crucial role in lowering the rates of illness and death caused by diseases that can be avoided.

The immune system serves as a crucial defence mechanism, safeguarding the body against pathogens via both innate and adaptive responses. It consists of multiple organs and immune cells that collaborate to detect and remove threats. Vaccination is essential for educating the immune system and ensuring enduring defence against infectious diseases. Grasping the intricacies of the immune system and recognising the critical role of vaccines is vital for advancing public health and thwarting disease outbreaks. By pursuing ongoing research and innovation, we can enhance our immune systems and secure a healthier future for everyone.

CHAPTER 11

The Integumentary System

The integumentary system represents the body's most extensive organ system, including the skin, hair, nails, and a variety of glands. It serves an essential function in safeguarding the organism, maintaining thermal balance, and enabling sensory awareness. This chapter delves into the intricate architecture and purpose of the skin, examining its various layers and functions, alongside the importance of hair, nails, and other skin appendages.

Skin: The Body's Shielding Layer

Strata of the Integument: Outer Layer, Middle Layer, Deep Layer

The skin is composed of three main layers, each serving unique functions and possessing specific characteristics:

1. Epidermis: The outermost layer of the skin, this layer is primarily made up of keratinised stratified squamous epithelium. This acts as the primary barrier against various environmental influences, including harmful microorganisms, toxic substances, and mechanical damage. The outer layer of skin possesses several important characteristics:

- Keratinocytes: These cells are the primary constituents of the epidermis, tasked with the production of keratin, a vital protective protein that aids in waterproofing the skin and minimising water loss.

- Melanocytes: Found in the basal layer of the epidermis, these cells are responsible for the production of melanin, which gives skin its colour. Melanin provides a degree of defence against detrimental ultraviolet (UV) radiation.

- Langerhans Cells: These specialised cells serve as vigilant guardians, identifying harmful invaders and initiating defensive mechanisms to safeguard the body from infections.

- Merkel Cells: These unique cells play a crucial role in sensory perception, especially in the detection of touch. These structures reside in the basal layer and establish connections with nerve endings.

The epidermis consists of five distinct layers, arranged from the outermost to the innermost: stratum corneum, stratum lucidum (which is found exclusively in thick skin), stratum granulosum, stratum spinosum, and stratum basale. Every layer plays a unique role in the intricate processes of skin renewal and defence.

2. Dermis: Located beneath the epidermis, the dermis is significantly thicker and plays a crucial role in providing structural support and elasticity to the skin. This structure is composed of connective tissue, blood vessels, lymphatic vessels, and nerve endings. The dermis consists of two primary layers:

- Papillary Layer: This upper layer is composed of loose connective tissue and features dermal papillae that interlock with the epidermis, strengthening the bond and expanding the surface area for nutrient exchange. This structure includes small blood vessels, lymphatic vessels, and sensory receptors that detect touch and pain sensations.

- Reticular Layer: This deeper section of the dermis consists of dense irregular connective tissue, which contributes to its strength and elasticity. This layer encompasses a significant number of skin structures, such as hair follicles, sebaceous glands, and sweat glands. The reticular layer is composed of collagen and elastin fibres, playing a crucial role in the skin's resilience and flexibility.

3. Subcutaneous Layer (Hypodermis): The subcutaneous layer represents the innermost stratum of the skin, primarily consisting of loose connective tissue and adipocytes, or fat cells. It fulfils multiple crucial roles:

- Insulation: The adipose layer serves to insulate the organism, preserving internal temperature and safeguarding the underlying musculature and organs from variations in temperature.

- Energy Storage: The adipose tissue functions as a reservoir of energy, supplying fuel for metabolic activities when required.

- Anchoring: The subcutaneous layer secures the skin to the structures beneath, including muscles and bones, while permitting a degree of movement.

Function of the Integumentary System in Defence, Sensory Perception, and Thermoregulation

The skin performs several essential roles, such as:

1. Protection: The skin serves as a vital shield against external dangers, encompassing microorganisms, harmful substances, and physical harm. The keratinised surface of the epidermis, along with the presence of antimicrobial peptides, plays a significant role in this

protective function. Furthermore, the skin plays a crucial role in minimising water loss, thereby aiding in the prevention of dehydration.

2. Sensation: The skin is equipped with a multitude of sensory receptors that respond to different stimuli, such as touch, pressure, pain, and temperature. These receptors play a crucial role in ensuring awareness of the surroundings and safeguarding the body from potential threats. The data collected by sensory receptors is relayed to the brain for analysis, facilitating suitable reactions to alterations in the environment.

3. Temperature Regulation: The skin is essential for maintaining body temperature through two primary mechanisms:

- Vasodilation and Vasoconstriction: The blood vessels within the dermis exhibit the ability to either dilate (widen) or constrict (narrow) as a reaction to fluctuations in temperature. In instances of elevated body temperature, there is a dilation of blood vessels, which enhances blood circulation to the surface of the skin, facilitating the dissipation of heat. On the other hand, in cold conditions, blood vessels narrow, leading to decreased blood flow to the skin and aiding in heat retention.

- Sweat Production: The glands located within the skin generate sweat, which then evaporates from the surface, leading to a cooling effect on the body. This mechanism plays a crucial role during exercise or in elevated temperatures.

Hair and Nails: Extensions of the Integumentary System

Role of Hair and Nails in the Organism

Hair and nails are regarded as extensions of the integumentary system, fulfilling several crucial roles:

1. Hair: The follicles, situated within the dermal layer, are responsible for generating hair strands that emerge from the surface of the skin. Hair performs multiple roles, such as:

- Protection: Hair serves as a barrier for delicate regions, including the eyes (eyelashes) and the scalp (head hair), safeguarding them from particles and ultraviolet rays.

- Sensation: Hair follicles are encircled by nerve endings, enabling the perception of light touch and variations in the environment. This sensory function serves to notify the organism of possible threats.

- Thermoregulation: The presence of hair can create a layer of trapped air near the skin, which serves as insulation and aids in maintaining body temperature. In certain species, fur plays a crucial role in preserving heat in frigid habitats.

2. Nails: Composed of resilient keratinised cells, nails play crucial protective and functional roles:

- Protection: Nails serve as a barrier for the tips of fingers and toes, increasing sensitivity and safeguarding the delicate tissues beneath from injury.

- Tool Use: Nails improve the capacity to hold and handle items, aiding in precise movements.

- Health Indicator: Alterations in nail appearance can signify a range of health issues. For instance, alterations in colour, fragility, or variations in form may indicate nutritional shortages or underlying health conditions.

Skin Appendages: Glands for Sweat and Oil Production

Skin appendages are essential for preserving skin health and supporting overall bodily functions:

1. Sweat Glands: The human body contains two primary categories of sweat glands:

- Eccrine Glands: These glands are found all over the body and play a crucial role in regulating body temperature. They generate a moisture-rich perspiration that aids in regulating body temperature via the process of evaporation.

- Apocrine Glands: Located primarily in certain regions like the armpits and groin, these glands produce a denser, milky secretion. During puberty, certain sweat glands become active, leading to the development of body odour due to the interaction of their secretions with skin bacteria.

2. Sebaceous Glands: These structures are linked to hair follicles and generate sebum, an oily secretion that aids in moisturising the skin and hair. Sebum serves multiple essential roles:

- Moisturization: Natural oils maintain hydration in the skin and hair, helping to avoid dryness and fragility.

- Antimicrobial Properties: Sebum comprises various compounds that exhibit antimicrobial characteristics, contributing to the skin's defence against infections.

- Barrier Function: By creating a delicate layer on the skin's surface, sebum improves the skin's barrier function, minimising water loss and blocking the entry of harmful substances.

The integumentary system represents a fascinating and vital aspect of the human body, consisting of the skin, hair, nails, and related glands. The skin functions as a crucial protective barrier, enhances sensory perception, and plays a key role in temperature regulation, whereas hair and nails fulfil both protective and functional purposes. Grasping the structure and functions of the integumentary system is essential for appreciating its significance in overall health and well-being. By implementing appropriate care and maintaining awareness, we can bolster the health of our skin and improve our body's capacity to defend against external dangers.

CHAPTER 12

The Reproductive System

The reproductive system plays a crucial role in ensuring the survival of species, enabling reproduction and the care of young organisms. It involves a sophisticated interaction of organs, hormones, and physiological mechanisms that facilitate gamete production, fertilisation, and gestation. This chapter will delve into the intricacies of the reproductive systems in both males and females, examining the roles of essential structures and the hormonal mechanisms that regulate reproduction.

Anatomy of Male and Female Reproductive Systems

Essential Components of Male and Female Reproductive Systems

The anatomical structures of the male and female reproductive systems are distinct, with each serving a crucial function in the process of reproduction.

Male Reproductive Anatomy:

1. Testes: The main reproductive organs in males, the testes play a crucial role in producing sperm and testosterone, which is the principal male sex hormone. Their position outside the body in the scrotum plays a crucial role in maintaining the appropriate temperature necessary for optimal sperm production.

2. Epididymis: This intricately coiled structure is positioned above each testis, functioning as a crucial

site for the maturation and storage of sperm cells. In this location, sperm acquire the ability to move and are retained until the moment of ejaculation.

3. Vas Deferens: A robust conduit responsible for the movement of sperm from the epididymis to the ejaculatory duct. It extends from the scrotum into the pelvic cavity, ultimately merging with the seminal vesicle.

4. Seminal Vesicles: These glands generate a substantial amount of the seminal fluid, providing nourishment to sperm and aiding in their movement. The fluid is composed of fructose and various other components that contribute to the well-being of sperm.

5. Prostate Gland: The prostate gland contributes additional fluid to the semen, incorporating enzymes and nutrients that play a crucial role in activating sperm. It additionally plays a role in the total quantity of semen produced.

6. Bulbourethral Glands (Cowper's Glands): These glands secrete a pre-ejaculatory fluid that aids in lubricating the urethra and counteracting any acidity from urine, creating a more favourable environment for sperm.

7. Penis: The external structure involved in reproduction, the penis facilitates the transfer of sperm into the female reproductive system. This structure comprises specialised tissue that fills with blood when stimulated, aiding in the process of penetration.

Female Reproductive System:

1. Ovaries: The female reproductive organs play a crucial role in generating ova (eggs) and secreting hormones like oestrogen and progesterone. Every female is endowed with a limited supply of eggs, which diminish in both quantity and quality as she ages.

2. Fallopian Tubes (Oviducts): These structures facilitate the movement of eggs from the ovaries to the uterus. Fertilisation generally takes place in the fallopian tubes, where the sperm encounters the egg.

3. Uterus: A hollow, muscular structure that serves as the site for implantation and development of a fertilised egg into a foetus. The uterus consists of three distinct layers: the endometrium, which serves as the inner lining; the myometrium, which is the muscular layer; and the perimetrium, which forms the outer layer.

4. Cervix: The lower segment of the uterus that connects to the vagina. It functions as a conduit for sperm to access the uterus and for menstrual fluid to leave the body. The cervix produces mucus that varies in consistency during the menstrual cycle, facilitating sperm transport.

5. Vagina: A muscular conduit linking the external reproductive structures to the uterus. The vagina functions as the passage for childbirth and is the site where sperm is introduced during sexual activity.

6. External Genitalia: Referred to as the vulva, this area encompasses various structures including the labia, clitoris, and vaginal opening. The clitoris is an intricate organ that significantly contributes to female sexual arousal.

Roles of Reproductive Structures in Propagation

The main role of the reproductive systems is to generate gametes (sperm in males and eggs in females), enable fertilisation, and nurture the growth of offspring.

- In male organisms, gametes are generated within the testes and subsequently stored in the epididymis. During ejaculation, sperm moves through the vas deferens, combines with seminal fluid from the seminal vesicles and prostate, and is released through the urethra.

- In females, the ovaries produce eggs during the process of ovulation, which are subsequently collected by the fallopian tubes. In the presence of sperm, the process of fertilisation may take place within the tubes. The fertilised egg journeys to the uterus, where it has the potential to implant in the endometrium and commence its development into a foetus.

Hormonal Control of Reproductive Processes

Influence of Hormones on Reproductive Cycles

Hormones are essential in managing the operations of the reproductive system in both males and females. These hormones are synthesised by different glands and operate through intricate feedback mechanisms.

1. In Males: - Testosterone: This hormone, mainly generated in the testes, plays a crucial role in the formation of male reproductive tissues, sperm production, and the emergence of secondary sexual traits (such as facial hair and a deeper voice).
- Luteinizing Hormone (LH) and Follicle-Stimulating Hormone (FSH): The hormones generated by the pituitary gland play a crucial role in stimulating

testosterone production and facilitating spermatogenesis within the testes.

2. In Females: - Oestrogen: Primarily synthesised in the ovaries, this hormone plays a vital role in the development of female reproductive tissues, the regulation of the menstrual cycle, and the support of pregnancy.
- Progesterone: Produced by the ovaries following ovulation, this hormone plays a crucial role in preparing the endometrium for implantation and sustaining pregnancy.
- Luteinizing Hormone (LH) and Follicle-Stimulating Hormone (FSH): These hormones produced by the pituitary gland play a crucial role in regulating the menstrual cycle, promoting the development of follicles and the process of ovulation.

Fundamentals of Fertilisation and Gestation

Fertilisation takes place when a sperm cell effectively enters an egg, resulting in the formation of a zygote. This procedure encompasses multiple essential stages:

1. Sperm Transport: Following ejaculation, sperm navigate through the vagina, cervix, and uterus, ultimately reaching the fallopian tubes, where they might meet an egg.

2. Capacitation: Prior to fertilisation, sperm experience a transformation known as capacitation, which improves their movement and capability to breach the egg's protective layers.

3. Fusion of Gametes: When a sperm meets an egg, it must navigate through its protective barriers (the corona radiata and zona pellucida). Upon the

penetration of the egg by a sperm, fertilisation takes place, leading to the merging of genetic material and the creation of a zygote.

4. Cell Division: The zygote experiences swift cell divisions while moving through the fallopian tube, resulting in the formation of a blastocyst. The duration of this process is approximately five to six days.

5. Implantation: The blastocyst reaches the uterus and embeds itself into the endometrium, marking the beginning of pregnancy. The process of successful implantation initiates hormonal shifts that sustain the uterine lining and inhibit the onset of menstruation.

6. Pregnancy Maintenance: Following implantation, the emerging placenta secretes hormones, such as human chorionic gonadotropin (hCG), which aids in sustaining the pregnancy and instructs the ovaries to persist in the production of oestrogen and progesterone.

7. Gestation: The duration of development from fertilisation to birth differs across species, with humans generally experiencing a gestation period of approximately 40 weeks. During this period, the growing foetus experiences remarkable changes and advancements, getting ready for existence beyond the womb.

The reproductive system comprises an intricate arrangement of organs and hormones that collaborate to enable the process of reproduction. Grasping the structure of the male and female reproductive systems, along with the hormonal control of reproduction, is essential for understanding the mechanisms that result in fertilisation and the emergence of new life. This understanding is essential for areas like healthcare, life sciences, and reproductive wellness, highlighting the significance of preserving reproductive health and being informed about reproductive options.

THE END

www.ingramcontent.com/pod-product-compliance
Lightning Source LLC
Chambersburg PA
CBHW070349230526
45471CB00006B/2489